I0412334

Table of Contents

Introduction

After years of dieting failures, constant hunger, and stubborn weight that just won't budge, you've finally decided you've had enough of the fad diets and constant deprivation. Like many people who've tried everything to get healthy and lose excess weight, it can be tough to figure out what the 'right' way of eating is. For years, we've been told that eating a diet high in healthy whole grains and low in saturated fat is the best way to get fit and avoid disease. Yet if this was true then why are so many of us still struggling with a spare tire, fatigue, and rising rates of heart disease, stroke, and diabetes?

This may come as a shock to you, but fat is not actually the bad guy it's been made out to be. In fact, fat can be the missing piece to supercharge your weight loss, balance your hormones, and give you long lasting energy! And that's why the ketogenic diet is so successful because it uses the power of healthy fats to get your body into a fat-burning state where magical things start to happen!

It may seem odd at first to skip the whole grain toast for the full-fat butter, but I can assure you that once you get the hang of creating your new fat-fuelled meals you'll never want to go back! No longer do you have to subsist off of dry and tasteless fare that leaves you fatigued and bloated. Now, you'll get to enjoy all of your favourite foods while leaning out and feeling great! You may be skeptical, thinking that this is just another fad diet that won't work in the long term, but nutritional ketosis is solidly backed by science and has a proven track record of helping people shed pounds and even treat chronic disease!

So if you are new to the ketogenic lifestyle, you've made the right decision by downloading this book! Everything you need to know about how to get started with a ketogenic diet can be found here including:

- How to fill your grocery cart with the most nutritious foods when you're at the grocery store.
- The benefits of being in ketosis including fat loss and improved memory!

- How to get your body into fat-burning mode more quickly!
- How to adapt the ketogenic diet to meet your unique needs.
- Tasty and easy keto-friendly recipes.
- And much more!

So don't wait another minute! Download this book today to learn more about getting started on the ketogenic diet!

Chapter 1: An Overview of the Ketogenic Diet

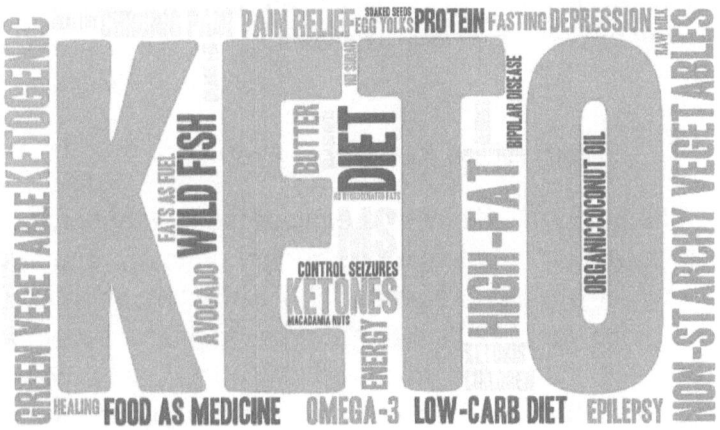

Before you can get started on a ketogenic diet, you need to know the science behind why it works, the benefits of being in nutritional ketosis, and who the diet is suitable for. Remember, knowledge is power, and if you know why the ketogenic diet is so effective then you're more likely to stick with it when you happen to be tempted by a plate of brownies!

What is the Ketogenic Diet?

First things first, what exactly is the ketogenic diet? As a beginner, you've probably seen plates of eggs and steak being consumed by friends, family, and coworkers who have already adopted this fat-fueled way of eating, but is the ketogenic diet really just about slamming back as much meat as possible? Not exactly. In fact, there's a bit more to the diet than simply eating as many animal products as you can stomach.

The ketogenic diet is a very low-carbohydrate and high-fat diet that includes moderate amounts of protein. By eating such a small amount of carbohydrates, you effectively put your body into a state called nutritional ketosis, which allows your body to use fat as fuel instead of glucose. Your body turns dietary and body fat into something called ketones, which your body can use as a source of fuel. Unlike other popular low-carb diets (e.g., The South Beach Diet), which tend to be high in protein, the ketogenic diet limits the amount of protein one eats to ensure the body stays in nutritional ketosis because eating excessive amounts of protein can actually prevent your body from using fat as fuel.

The Origin of the Ketogenic Diet

The ketogenic diet isn't the latest fad diet that promises to melt your fat away, only to leave you hungry, irritated, and ten pounders heavier than when you started. In fact, the ketogenic diet has been around since the 1920's when it was originally developed to treat epilepsy. Originally, the diet was developed as a way to provide patients with the benefits that come from fasting. In fact, dating back to 1911, doctors were experimenting with using fasting as a therapeutic modality for treating patient's epilepsy. The only problem was that it was impossible to fast indefinitely (obviously), so once the patients began to eat again, their seizures would return.

But in 1921 a doctor named Rollin Woodyatt discovered that molecules produced by the liver during starvation (acetone, beta-hydroxybutyrate, and acetoacetate) were also produced when a person ate a diet high in fat and low in carbohydrates. This high-fat diet was officially termed the 'ketogenic diet' by Russel Wilder in 1921, who used it as a treatment for epilepsy. The diet was effective at eliminating patients' seizures, but eventually fell out of favour as new anticonvulsant medications were developed. Nevertheless, the ketogenic diet is still an effective treatment therapy for epilepsy, and is especially effective for children.[1]

Nutritional Ketosis 101

Are You A Sugar Burner or a Fat Burner?

You know that being in ketosis means burning fat for fuel instead of sugar, but maybe you'd like to know a bit more about the biology behind how ketosis actually occurs in our bodies. The first thing you should know is that most people are 'sugar burners', which means their bodies run off of glucose as a source of fuel. Whenever you eat carbohydrates or too much protein, you're supplying your body with the materials it needs to create glucose. Glucose can be used as a source of immediate energy (e.g., running to catch the bus) or stored in the liver and muscles as glycogen to be used as energy in the future.

Depending on how much muscle mass you have, your body should be able to store anywhere from 1000-1600 calories of glucose as energy before it has to resort to using other forms of fuel when you run out. This is why we see long distance runners and bikers 'carbing up' the night before a big event in an effort to fill their muscles with as much glycogen as possible before a big race! But if our bodies do run out of glucose, it needs another source of fuel it can use in an emergency. And this is where nutritional ketosis enters the equation because using fat as a fuel source is something our bodies have been doing for as long as humans have been around.

You see, back in our hunter-gatherer days, there were often times when we had to go for periods of time without food. Hunter-gatherers didn't really have the luxury of 24/7 grocery stores, so it could be days before they saw their next meal. And during these periods of 'semi-starvation', it was essential that our ancestors could use their body fat reserves as a source of fuel or else the human race would have become extinct pretty quickly!

The Science Behind Ketosis

Therefore, you don't have to worry about nutritional ketosis as being 'unnatural' or 'dangerous' because humans have been doing it for as long as we've existed on this planet! Being in nutritional ketosis means our bodies are using ketones, derived from fat, as a source of fuel instead of glucose. And compared to the relatively small supply of glucose we store in our livers and muscles as glycogen, our bodies have access to a much larger supply of ketones in the form of body fat! This is why monks and spiritual gurus can fast for such long periods of time without experiencing any negative health consequences because they are literally living off of their body fat reserves. In fact, the longest fast ever undertaken lasted 382 days, and the only 'food' the patient consumed were vitamins and electrolytes. This particular man lost 276 pounds over the course of his fast, and was under the medical supervision of a doctor.[2] Although most people don't have the body fat reserves to survive for more than a year not eating any food, this man does provide a good example of how our bodies can function and even thrive by converting fat into ketones through the process of ketosis.

And by adopting a ketogenic diet, you're effectively mimicking the same processes the body undertakes when you fast. A diet that is very low in carbohydrates and high in fat forces your body to switch from burning glucose to ketones as fuel. As our blood sugar and insulin levels drop from a reduction in carbohydrates, stored and dietary fat is made accessible as a fuel source. Then, a hormone called hormone-sensitive lipase breaks down this fat into fatty acid molecules and a glycerol molecule. The fatty acids are transported to your mitochondria (little energy factories inside of every cell) where they are used in a process called 'beta-oxidation'. One of the end products of beta-oxidation is acetyl-CoA, a molecule that is used in the process we know as ketogenesis.

Now this is where the magic happens. During ketogenesis, acetyl-CoA is converted into ketone bodies (acetone, acetoacetate, and beta-hydroxybutyrate). As the level of ketones in the blood rises, the body and brain start using them as a source of fuel. Maintain a low carbohydrate and high fat diet, and you will be able to keep your body in a permanent state of ketosis where your body runs off of fat (aka. ketones) instead of glucose.

Is Ketosis Safe?

You may still have some hesitations about being in ketosis. Maybe you've done a bit of research on the internet and came across the term 'diabetic ketoacidosis', which is a condition that can be deadly! But just to be clear, there is a difference between diabetic ketoacidosis and nutritional ketosis.

Nutritional ketosis is a completely safe and natural state to be in. As mentioned previously, our hunter-gatherer ancestors were probably in a state of ketosis quite often as food supplies dwindled. You can enter a state of nutritional ketosis by fasting or by eating a high-fat and low-carb ketogenic diet. In contrast, diabetic ketoacidosis is a condition that can occur in type 1 diabetics if they don't take enough insulin, and is the result of excessive ketone production in the body. Symptoms of diabetic ketoacidosis include vomiting, abdominal pain, confusion, coma, and even death. If someone is experiencing diabetic ketoacidosis, they need to seek medical attention immediately.

So although the production of ketones are involved in both nutritional ketosis and diabetic ketoacidosis, they are not one and the same. The concentration of ketones in the blood of someone in nutritional ketosis never rises higher than 3 millimolar/L. Even if you fasted for a week, your blood ketones likely wouldn't rise higher than 6 or 7 millimolar/L. In contrast, the blood ketone levels of someone in diabetic ketoacidosis occurs at a minimum of 10 millimolar/L. Therefore, as long as you aren't a type I diabetic and your pancreas is producing sufficient quantities of insulin, then it would be extremely difficult, if not impossible, to experience ketoacidosis. This is because the pancreas will secrete insulin in response to high levels of ketones to create a feedback loop to tell the body to stop producing anymore ketones.

Chapter 2: Is the Ketogenic Diet Right For Me?

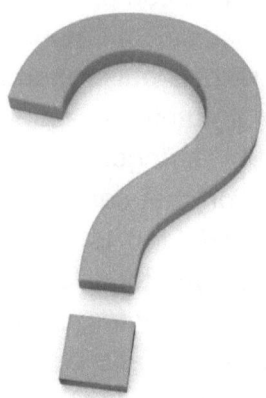

Check out some of the benefits of switching to a ketogenic diet below! In addition to helping you burn fat and get fit, being in nutritional ketosis can improve a number of chronic conditions! At the same time, ensure that you don't fall into any of the categories of people who a ketogenic diet potentially wouldn't be safe for. We're all unique individuals, and just because a diet works for someone else doesn't necessarily mean it's the best diet for you.

Benefits of the Ketogenic Diet

Burn Fat & Lose Weight: Being in ketosis has been shown to increase your metabolism, control fat-storing insulin levels, and keep you satiated so you won't spend your evenings snacking on chips and chocolate bars. The result is a body that wants to burn fat and build lean muscle! In fact, studies have demonstrated that a high-fat diet consistently outperforms the conventional healthy whole grains low-fat diet that is routinely recommended by healthcare practitioners. Participants typically lose 2.2-3x more weight following a ketogenic diet during these studies! [3,4]

Increase Brain Power: By getting your brain to use ketones for fuel instead of glucose, you'll be boosting your brainpower for better memory, attention, and focus! Eating a ketogenic diet is even being used to treat a variety of neurologic conditions including Parkinson's, ALS, severe depression, autism, Alzheimer's, and chronic migraines. [5,6]

Treat Heart Disease: New research is showing that excessive carbohydrate consumption is actually the main trigger for atherosclerosis and elevated triglyceride levels! But adopting a high-fat and low-carb diet can result in a drop in blood triglycerides, LDL 'bad' cholesterol levels, while increasing HDL 'good' cholesterol levels. [7,8]

Treat Type 2 Diabetes: Type 2 diabetes can be characterized as a combination of high blood sugar, insulin resistance (where the cells don't respond to insulin), and an overall lack of insulin. While genetics may make someone more susceptible to developing type 2 diabetes, lifestyle and diet can be used to effectively control and even reverse the condition. A ketogenic diet has been shown to improve insulin sensitivity by 75%, helping sufferers get off diabetes medication and lose weight! [9,10]

Treat Cancer: The ketogenic diet has even been used to effectively treat cancer (in addition to alternative and conventional healing recommendations). Being in a state of nutritional ketosis is effective against fast-growing cancer cells because cancer cells are sugar eaters. In fact, cancer cells have ten times as many insulin receptors on their cell membrane that a regular cell does. And all of those insulin receptors are there to escort glucose, cancer cells' favourite food, into the cell where it can be used as energy. By cutting off cancer's favourite food supply, you're also preventing cancer from growing. In fact, a ketogenic diet has been shown to be especially effective at reducing the growth of brain tumours. [11,12]

People Who Should Not Be in Ketosis

Although being in a state of nutritional ketosis is safe, the ketogenic diet may not be optimal for everyone. You may want to speak to your doctor if you fall into any of the following categories.

Are You On Medication? : Being on a ketogenic diet can affect how your body metabolizes medications and can alter their effects. Dieters may experience a sudden decrease in blood pressure if they're on blood pressure medication, a decrease in blood sugar if they're using insulin to manage diabetes, or cause a concentration of lithium for those who have a mental health condition. It's always best to speak with your doctor before you start a ketogenic diet to ensure you won't be interfering with the effects of your medication.

Do You Have a Gallbladder? : The gallbladder is important for helping the body digest fats, so if you had this organ removed (or it's diseased) then you'll have a difficult time adjusting to a high-fat diet.

Have You Had Bariatric Surgery? : Weight loss surgery alters the size of the stomach or makes it more difficult for your small intestine to absorb nutrients. Undergoing such a procedure will make it more difficult for you to absorb fats and get proper nutrition from a ketogenic diet.

Are You Pregnant or Breastfeeding? : Your protein needs will likely be higher than what is provided on a ketogenic diet.

Are You a Child? : Protein requirements tend to be higher in younger people, and can vary by age as well.

Do You Have a Tendency to Get Kidney Stones? : Going on a ketogenic diet could cause the formation of kidney stones since the diet tends to alter salt and water balance.

Are You Very Thin? : One of the many reasons people start a ketogenic diet is to drop extra weight, so if you're already thin then you may want to a) increase your fat intake or b) increase your carbohydrate intake so you're not in ketosis all the time to avoid losing too much weight.

People Who Would Benefit From Ketosis

Do You Have Type 2 Diabetes?: While type 1 diabetics need to be a bit more cautious about starting a ketogenic diet because their pancreases may produce insufficient insulin, type 2 diabetics can experience vast benefits from adopting a ketogenic diet because it will lower their blood glucose and improve insulin sensitivity.

Are You Overweight or Obese?: By switching into nutritional ketosis, you are helping your body access body fat as a source of fuel. Also, many people who struggle with weight loss also happen to be insulin resistant, which this diet will also rectify.

Do You Struggle With a Mood Disorder?: There is some evidence that eating a ketogenic diet could help treat mood disorders, such as bipolarism, by increasing energy to the brain.

Do You Have Cardiovascular Disease?: Mounting evidence is demonstrating that excessive carbohydrate intake rather than fat is the real cause of atherosclerosis and plaque buildup in the arteries. Eating a high-fat and low-carb diet can actually reduce 'bad' cholesterol and one's chances of suffering a heart attack.

And these are just a few types of people who could benefit from a ketogenic diet. In fact, just check out the full list of benefits below for what you can expect to experience from going on a ketogenic diet.

Chapter 3: How to Get Started on a Ketogenic Diet

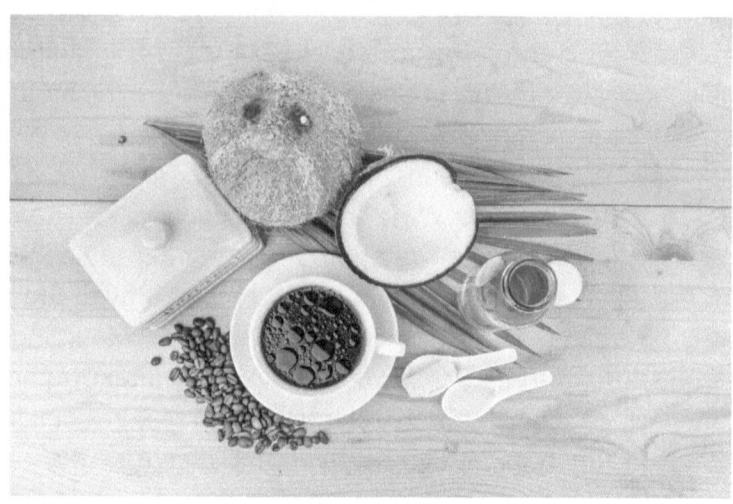

So you've officially decided you want to take the plunge into a ketogenic diet. I can promise you that you won't be disappointed! But as a beginner to nutritional ketosis, you may be confused about how to start. Do you need to throw out everything in your fridge and pantries? Should you be eating lard by the spoonful, while avoiding anything that isn't a piece of meat? These are all good questions, and need to be answered if you want to do 'keto' right. And the first step before you can get started on a ketogenic diet is to make sure that your kitchen is full of keto-friendly foods. So the next time you go to the grocery store, take this list with you to ensure you're buying foods that will make you a fat-burner!

Keto-Friendly Food List

Meat: Chicken, Turkey, and Beef.

Note: This is not the time to buy skinless and lean cuts of meat. Remember, the ketogenic diet is a high fat diet, so choose fattier cuts of meat like chicken thighs and well marbled beef! Also, try to buy organic and free-range meat if possible. Many conventional forms of meat are full of antibiotics and hormones that can disrupt your own hormonal balance.

Fatty Fish: Salmon, Herring, Sardines, Sablefish, Trout, Tuna, Mackerel, and Swordfish.

Note: Try to buy sustainably caught fish to ensure you're not contributing to the reduction of an endangered species. Also, consider eating smaller fish like sardines because they will not have accumulated as many of the pollutants that are now in our seas (e.g., mercury). Large fish like tuna are more likely to contain high levels of ocean contaminants from industrial pollution.

Eggs: Chicken, Duck, Quail.

Note: Prioritize free-range and organic.

High-Fat Dairy: Butter, Cream, Cheese.

Note: Many people cannot tolerate dairy, so it's not mandatory to eat dairy on a ketogenic diet. If you can tolerate dairy then ensure you're buying organic and pasture-fed products.

Nuts & Seeds: Almonds, Macadamia Nuts, Walnuts, Flaxseeds, Pumpkin Seeds, Chia Seeds.

Healthy Oils: Extra Virgin Olive Oil, Coconut Oil, Avocado Oil

Low-Sugar Fruit: Avocados, Lemons, Limes, Berries

Note: Berries should be eaten sparingly. It's best to avoid most fruit while you're trying to get into ketosis. Save the sweeter fare for later when you're solidly in a ketogenic state.

Low-Carbohydrate Vegetables: Green vegetables (leafy greens, broccoli, cucumber, cabbage etc.), Tomatoes, Onions, Peppers, Cauliflower, Mushrooms, Zucchini.

Condiments: Pepper, Salt, Herbs, Mustard, Mayonnaise (that doesn't contain canola oil).

Beverages: Coffee, Tea

Note: prioritize organic and free trade.

Avoid These Foods

Avoid picking up any of these foods on your next shopping trip. And if you already have them at home in your pantry, consider giving them away to friends, family, or a charitable organization so they won't go to waste.

Processed and Packaged Foods: Cereals, Cakes, Sodas, Juices, Ice Cream, Candy.

Note: Try to avoid buying anything in the inner aisles of the grocery store, and stick to the perimeter where you'll find fresh produce, meats, and dairy.

Grains & Pseudo-Grains: Oats, Wheat, Rye, Barley, Spelt, Rice, Quinoa, Amaranth, Freekeh etc.

Note: Also, avoid the products made from these grains including cereal, oatmeal, granola bars, bread, and baked goods.

High-Carbohydrate Vegetables: Potatoes, Yams, Carrots, Turnips, Parsnips, Peas, Corn, Yucca.

Legumes: All Beans Including Kidney Beans, Navy Beans, Chickpeas, Mung Beans, Lentils, and Peanuts.

Fruit: Avoid All Fruit

Note: Lemons, limes, avocados, and berries being notable exceptions.

Condiments: BBQ Sauce, Ketchup, Conventional Salad Dressings, Honey, Maple Syrup, and Agave Nectar.

Note: Check the label of any condiment you buy. Most have high levels of carbohydrates from added sugar.

Unhealthy Fats: Canola Oil, Soybean Oil, Corn Oil.

Note: These oils are highly inflammatory and are found in many processed and packaged foods.

Alcohol: Wine, Beer, Coolers, Gin, Whisky etc.

Note: The carbohydrate content in many alcoholic drinks can prevent the body from entering and staying in ketosis.

The Ideal Macronutrient Ratio

Now that you've got a fridge full of keto-friendly foods to make your next delicious fat-fueled dish, you need to know how to structure your meals to ensure you're getting enough fat, and not too many carbohydrates or protein. Follow this macronutrient ratio to ensure your meals are keto-approved!

As a general rule of thumb, the fewer carbohydrates you eat, the easier it will be to enter and stay in ketosis. Most people need to eat fewer than 50g of carbs per day to stay in ketosis, while eating under 20g of carbohydrates is said to be optimal. The ideal macronutrient ratio on a ketogenic diet is 10% of calories coming from carbohydrates, 15-25% coming from protein, and 70% or more coming from fat. In the beginning, you'll probably have to use a tracking device like **Cronometer** or **My Fitness Pal** to ensure your meals are close to replicating these ratios. But over time, you'll find that you develop a knack for accurately estimating the macronutrient content of your meals, and how to ensure you don't eat too much protein or carbohydrates.

Chapter 4: How to Get Into Ketosis

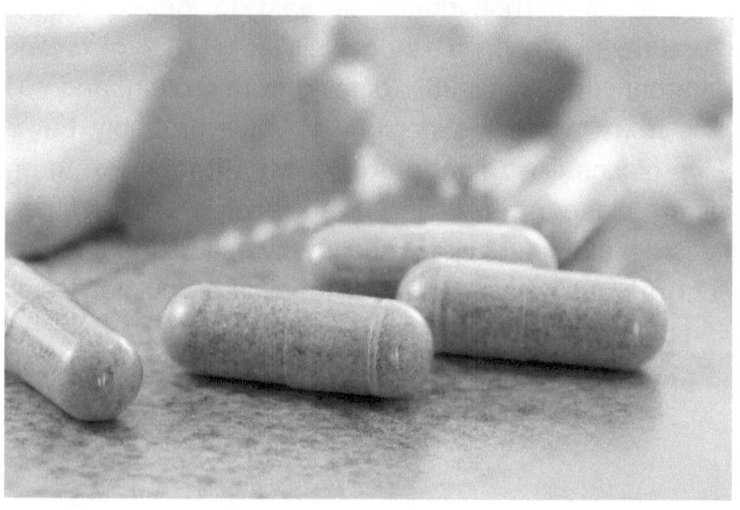

The entire point of a ketogenic diet is to turn your body into a fat burner instead of a sugar burner. You want to be in the state called nutritional ketosis, which is where your body is turning to ketones for fuel instead of glucose. But how does one get into ketosis? Is eating the ketogenic diet enough to kickstart your body's fat burning potential? It's true that following the ketogenic diet will eventually shift your metabolic state to where you're burning ketones for energy instead of glucose, but this can take longer than what most people are willing to wait for. We do tend to be creatures of immediate gratification after all! But pairing your ketogenic diet with these supplement and lifestyle modifications will push you into ketosis faster and more efficiently! So give them a try today!

Ketosis-Promoting Dietary Suggestions

Limit Carbohydrates: When you first start the ketogenic diet, it's important to restrict your carbohydrates to 20g or less a day. Although you may be able to maintain ketosis on a higher number of carbohydrates, it's important during the beginning that you limit carbs. In the beginning, limit or completely avoid all fruit and vegetables with higher carbohydrate levels (even onions and tomatoes). Once in ketosis, you can reintroduce some of these higher carbohydrate foods that are still keto-friendly.

Limit Protein: Many ketogenic dieters make the mistake of thinking they can eat as much protein as they want because it's not a carbohydrate. Unfortunately, eat too much protein and your body will turn the excess into glucose, effectively kicking your body out of ketosis. Avoid buying lean cuts of meat like skinless chicken breast, shellfish, and turkey, which tend to be high in protein, but low in fat.

Eat Enough Fat: Don't be fat-phobic because this diet requires that you embrace healthy fats! Ensure you're getting at least 70% of your calories from fats. If you're having trouble eating enough fat, turn to easily digested and condensed forms of fat like nut butters and coconut oil.

Try Intermittent Fasting: Try limiting your meals to a 4-8 hour time window. The break your body will get from not constantly eating will help boost ketone levels and shift your body into ketosis sooner. Remember, everyone is different and fasting works better for some people than others. Women have the tendency to experience hormonal imbalance if they fast for too long, so either reduce your fasting window or avoid fasting altogether if you start to notice issues with your thyroid, stress levels, or menstrual cycle.

Try a Fat Fast: For a period of 2-4 days, you'll be eating 90% fat spread out between 3-4 meals throughout the day. You can eat foods like macadamia nuts, egg yolks, canola oil-free mayonnaise, bulletproof coffee (organic coffee with butter/MCT oil/coconut oil). Avoid doing a fat fast longer than five days or else your body will start to break down muscle tissue.

Avoid Snacking Between Meals: Snacking will reduce ketone levels in the blood, so it's best to eat until satiety at each meal and avoid snacking in between.

Eat More Coconut Oil: Coconut oil is unique in the sense that it is not stored by the body. Instead, it's rapidly used for energy and increases your body's metabolic rate.

Ketosis-Promoting Exercise

Combining a low carbohydrate diet with exercise will more quickly deplete your carbohydrate reserves (aka. glycogen). And when you run out of glycogen, your liver will start using body fat to provide you with energy, effectively shifting your body into ketosis.

The best exercises for getting into a ketogenic state include high-intensity exercise because this type of activity relies heavily on muscle glycogen for fuel.

- Sprinting
- High Speed Cycling
- Any Form of Fasted Cardio (aka. Where you refrain from eating before a workout session to more effectively drain muscle and liver glycogen)
- HIIT (High Intensity Interval Training)
- Circuit Training
- Heavy Resistance Training

Try this glycogen-depleting full-body workout to speed your transition into ketosis!

Glycogen-Depleting Workout

- Leg Press: 2 sets, 10-15 reps
- Barbell Bench Press: 2 sets, 10-15 reps
- Seated Cable Rows: 2 sets, 10-15 reps
- Barbell Shoulder Press: 2 sets, 10-15 reps
- Barbell Lunge: 2 sets, 10-15 reps
- Lat Pulldown: 2 sets, 10-15 reps
- Standing Calf Raises: 2 sets, 10--15 reps
- Dumbbell Bicep Curl: 2 sets, 10-15 reps
- Pushups: 2 sets, 10-15 reps
- Hanging Leg Raise: 2 sets, 10-15 reps

Note: To more effectively deplete your glycogen levels, you want to train till 'failure', which means using the highest possible weights (or 'loads') for each set of reps.

Ketosis-Promoting Supplements

Exogenous Ketones: By providing your body with ketones in the form of a supplement, you can enter ketosis faster and/or be more flexible with your diet. Exogenous ketones can allow you to eat more carbohydrates and less fat than you normally would while trying to enter or maintain ketosis.

MCT Oil: A source of medium-chain triglycerides, MCT oil enters your cells' mitochondria and allows your body to easily and quickly produce ketones without excessive effort. In comparison to other fats like omega-3s, the body must utilize a more extensive and complicated process to turn these fats into ketones.

How to Know When You're In Ketosis

So now that you're doing everything you can to get into nutritional ketosis, how will you actually know when you've made the transition from burning glucose as fuel to fat?

Symptoms of Ketosis

- **Increased Frequency of Urination:** Shifting into ketosis can cause increased urination. At the same time, you can also test for ketone bodies using urine strips. The only caveat is that these strips can be expensive, and many dieters prefer to rely on symptoms instead of constantly checking their ketone levels with strips.

- **Increased Thirst and Dry Mouth:** Peeing more often will also result in increased thirst (since you're dehydrating your body) and dry mouth.

- **'Keto' Breath:** Your breath may smell fruity or like fermented fruit as a result of ketone bodies in your breath. This interesting odour is usually temporary.

- **Less Hunger:** There are a number of causes of increased satiation (e.g., fat is more filling than carbohydrates), but one potential cause is your body accessing body fat to use as fuel when it switches into ketosis.

- **More Energy:** After experiencing the 'keto flu' for the first couple of days or weeks, your body will become fat-adapted and you'll experience a marked improvement in energy and focus.

Using Ketone Strips to Measure Ketosis

If you do want to use ketone strips to test your urine for ketone bodies, you'll need to know the ranges for what is considered optimal ketosis. When you use ketosis strips you're actually measuring acetoacetate, a type of ketone body. Anywhere from 1.5-3.0 mmol/L is considered optimal for maximum mental and physical well being including fat-burning and weight loss. Going above 3 mmol/L won't necessarily give you better results, and higher levels can sometimes be an indication you're in a state of semi-starvation due to severe calorie restriction. Being between 0.5-1.5 mmol/L is considered light nutritional ketosis. You will start to experience some of the benefits of being in fat-burning mode at these levels, but it isn't.

Enjoying this book so far? I'd love it for you to share your thoughts and post a quick review on Amazon!

Chapter 5: Making the Ketogenic Diet Work for You

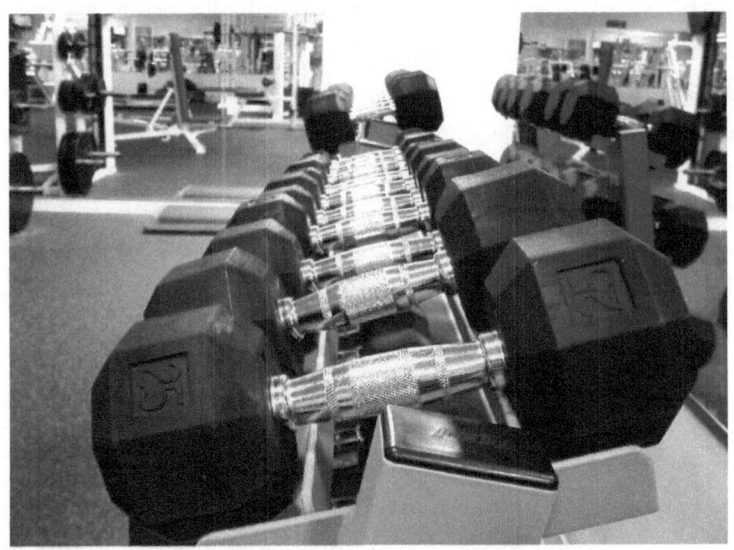

Did you know that there is more than one way to do the ketogenic diet? It's true! There are certain categories of people, including athletes and women, who may find that adding some slight modifications to the standard ketogenic diet can improve the results they experience and their performance at the gym. In addition to the standard ketogenic diet, there are two other subtypes including the cyclical ketogenic diet and the targeted ketogenic diet.

The Standard Ketogenic Diet

As a refresher, the standard ketogenic diet is adhering to the macronutrient ratio outlined in Chapter 3 where fat is 75% of your caloric intake, protein is 20%, and carbohydrates are 5%. Dieters will adhere to this macronutrient ratio at every meal to ensure their bodies stay in nutritional ketosis.

The Cyclical Ketogenic Diet

A cyclical ketogenic diet combines a low-carbohydrate diet with periods of higher carbohydrate consumption. These periods of eating a larger number of carbohydrates are called 'refeeds' where dieters focus on eating healthy carbs like sweet potatoes, starchy vegetables, and fruits. The carbohydrates from these foods will fill up liver and muscle glycogen stores. And because muscle and liver glycogen was depleted from being on a low-carb diet, the carbohydrates consumed will solely be used to replenish these stores and not stored as body fat. You may notice a small weight gain after a refeed, but this is usually all water and not body fat.

People Who Would Benefit from a Cyclical Ketogenic Diet:

- Endurance Athletes: Carbohydrate refeeds will refill liver and muscle glycogen, which is necessary for optimal performance for athletes, especially those engaged in endurance activities.
- Athletes Looking to Bulk: Having periods of high carbohydrate consumption makes it easier for your body to put on mass.

In terms of how many refeed days you need and how many carbohydrates you'll need to eat, it will be fairly individual. The standard protocol for following a cyclical ketogenic diet includes 5-6 days of low-carbohydrate eating and 1-2 days of high-carb eating. You could also try going longer periods without carbs (10-12 days), and then refeeding for 4-5 days.

The Cyclical Ketogenic Diet for Athletes

If you're interested in a cyclical diet because you want to optimize your performance as an athlete, you need to schedule your workouts so that you're completely depleting your muscle glycogen during your high carb refeed days. To undertake a carb refeed properly, try to adhere to this plan:

Day 1: Eat a macronutrient ratio of 70% carbohydrates, 15% protein, and 15% fats with a focus on high glycemic index carbohydrates like oatmeal, pasta, corn, potatoes, carrots, and sweet fruits.

Day 2: Eat a macronutrient ratio of 60% carbohydrates, 25% protein, and 15% fats with a focus on low glycemic carbohydrates like legumes, nuts, pseudo grains (quinoa, amaranth), and low-sugar fruits including plums, apples, oranges, and pears).

These two days of high carbohydrate eating are the perfect times to schedule your high-intensity cardio or weight lifting workouts. On Day 2 of your carb refeed, try to schedule your last workout five hours after your last meal of the day. After your two days of high carb eating, you simply switch to a standard ketogenic diet for the next five days until your next carb refeed.

How to Get Back Into Ketosis After a Carb Refeed?

The best way to re-enter ketosis after a carb refeed is to perform a glycogen-depleting workout on an empty stomach the day after your carb refeed ends. HIIT (high intensity interval training) or an intense weight training session are great options for depleting muscle and liver glycogen. Also, sticking to lower glycemic carbohydrate choices will make it easier for your body to re-enter ketosis, so skip the sugar-laden cereals and candy bars, and stick with healthier options like sweet potatoes, beans, and whole grains during your refeeds. Also, the longer you've been on the ketogenic diet, the easier it will be for you to re-enter ketosis after a carb refeed.

The Targeted Ketogenic Diet

The targeted ketogenic diet is simply a standard ketogenic diet with the addition of carbohydrates around your workouts or other specific time periods. The targeted ketogenic diet may actually be a better choice for most people, especially beginners, who may have trouble reentering ketosis after a huge carb refeed. By selectively eating carbs around your workouts, you'll minimize the time your body spends out of ketosis because you should be depleting your muscle and liver glycogen during your workouts, so that your body won't revert to burning glucose instead of fat for longer periods of time.

People Who Would Benefit From a Targeted Ketogenic Diet

- Active Dieters (especially those engaged in anaerobic activity like weightlifting)
- Women and those prone to hormonal imbalances: Women's hormone levels tend to be more sensitive to extremely low carbohydrate diets, so including a small amount of carbohydrates can be helpful in increasing leptin levels to upregulate hormones and thyroid production.

The Targeted Ketogenic Diet for Active Dieters

Many people who are involved in weightlifting or other forms of anaerobic exercise state that they experience better performance if they precede their workout with the consumption of carbohydrates. If you do want to do a small carb up before a workout, most dieters find that 25-50g of carbohydrates 30 minutes before a workout is sufficient for optimal performance.

And because you want these mini carb ups to be used as instant energy for your current workout, it's best to focus on high glycemic carb sources like white potatoes, white bread, corn, carrots, white rice, honey, and maple syrup that will be quickly absorbed as glucose into the bloodstream. You may drop out of ketosis for a few hours after your workout due to higher insulin levels, but as the blood glucose is absorbed into your muscles and liver to replenish glycogen levels you'll re-enter ketosis quite easily. As a rule of thumb, try to avoid foods high in fructose, which is absorbed by the liver and can prevent the body from quickly reentering ketosis after your workout.

The Targeted Ketogenic Diet for Hormone Balance

As a good rule of thumb, if you're someone suffering from hormonal imbalance, it's a good idea to have a small carb refeed every night to reduce your cortisol (stress) levels and improve the function of your thyroid. In terms of how many carbs you should include in a refeed, it will vary depending on your own individual constitution and how out of balance your hormones are. If you're just starting to incorporate a small refeed every night then try a ratio of 50% carbohydrates, 25% protein, and 25% fat and adjust accordingly.

Other Suggestions for Balancing Hormones

- Reduce Exercise Intensity
- Ensure You're Getting Adequate Sleep
- Reduce Stress Levels (meditation, journaling, yoga)
- Avoid Endocrine-Disrupting Toxins (found in conventional personal care products, conventional meat and dairy)

The Vegan Ketogenic Diet

Whether you're a vegan for health reasons, or you are a staunch ethical vegan who doesn't believe in eating any animal-derived products, it is still possible for you to gain the benefits from following a ketogenic diet! No, you won't be eating platefuls of butter and beef, but there are many plant-based sources of fat you can use to get your body into nutritional ketosis. It may be a bit more difficult to attain the prescribed macronutrient ratio recommended for a standard ketogenic diet (75/20/5), but it definitely is still possible to get your body into a fat-burning state on a plant-based diet.

Vegan Fat Sources

- Avocado Oil and Avocados
- Cocoa Butter
- Coconut Oil*
- Flaxseed Oil
- Macadamia Oil
- MCT Oil*
- Olive Oil
- Coconut Cream
- Olives

Note: * Coconut and MCT oil are excellent sources of medium-chain fats that help the body burn fat for energy instead of glucose, so eat these oils in abundance to get your body into nutritional ketosis.

Vegan Protein Sources

- Tofu
- Pumpkin Seeds
- Almonds/Almond Flour
- Flaxseed
- Chia Seeds
- Brazil Nuts
- Hazelnuts
- Walnuts
- Pecans
- Macadamia Nuts
- Coconut

Vegan Low-Carbohydrate Vegetables

- All Lettuces (e.g., romaine, spinach, endive, arugula etc.)
- Celery
- Collard Greens
- Eggplant
- Asparagus
- Radishes
- Tomatoes
- Cucumber
- Cauliflower
- Broccoli
- Bell Pepper
- Cabbage
- Fennel
- Mushrooms
- Green Beans
- Bok Choy

Chapter 6: Keto-Friendly Recipes

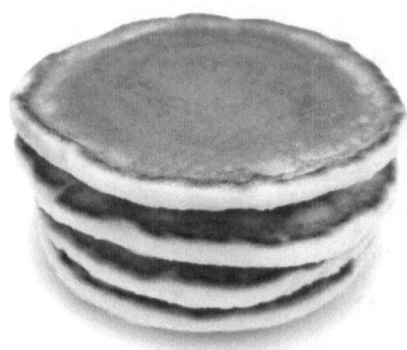

Maybe you're sick of eggs, or you just want to switch up your routine a bit. Try some of these delicious fat-fueled recipes that are keto-friendly.

Breakfast

Baked Egg in Turkey Cups

The perfect breakfast for when you're on the run! Simply grab a few of these baked egg in turkey cups for a quick and tasty morning meal!

Ingredients:
- 6 eggs
- 12 pieces of thinly sliced turkey deli slices
- 3 tbsp of diced scallions
- Optional: shredded cheddar cheese

Directions:
1. Preheat oven to 400 degrees Fahrenheit
2. Grease muffin tins with coconut oil or butter.

3. Fit two slices of turkey into each muffin cup to form a makeshift bowl.
4. Crack an egg into the turkey-lined muffin tin.
5. Top with scallions and optional cheese if you prefer.
6. Bake for 15-20 minutes.

Enjoy!

Keto-Friendly 'Porridge'

Sometimes it can be nice to treat yourself to a warm bowl of porridge, especially as the temperatures drop. Fortunately, this porridge is keto-friendly and full of healthy plant-based fats!

Ingredients:
- 2 tbsp chia seed
- 2 tbsp ground flaxseed
- ½ cup almond milk
- ½ tsp cinnamon
- Optional Toppings: low-sugar berries, coconut oil or coconut butter

Directions:
1. Add chia seed, ground flaxseed, and almond milk in a saucepan and bring to boil over medium heat.
2. Stir frequently. The porridge will thicken quickly. When it does, remove from heat.
3. Add toppings.

Enjoy!

Almond Flour Pancakes

A great breakfast for lazy Sunday mornings. These pancakes are delicious and will keep your body in a fat-burning state.

Ingredients:

- ½ cup almond flour
- ¼ tsp salt
- ½ tsp baking powder
- 1 egg
- ¼ tsp vanilla extract
- ½ tbsp heavy whipping cream
- Optional: Coconut oil, butter, or nut butters

Directions:
1. Preheat a frying pan at low to medium heat.
2. Mix together almond flour, salt, and baking powder in a bowl.
3. In a separate bowl, mix together egg, vanilla extract, and heavy whipping cream.
4. Mix wet and dry ingredients together.
5. Add butter or coconut oil to frying pan, and spoon batter into the pan. Flip pancakes when underside is a golden brown colour.
6. Optional: Top with coconut butter, butter, nut butter, or coconut oil.

Enjoy!

Main Meals

Avocado Egg Boats

This simple meal is bound to impress with its presentation, but preparing it couldn't be any easier!

Ingredients:
- 1 avocado
- 2 eggs
- 1 tbsp of cheddar cheese

Directions:
1. Preheat oven to 425 degrees Fahrenheit.
2. Cut avocado in half and remove the pit.
3. Using a spoon, make a wider indent in each half of the avocado so it will comfortably hold an egg. Place each avocado half in a muffin tin.
4. Crack an egg in each avocado.
5. Cook for 15 minutes.

Enjoy!

Keto-Friendly Bread

Who said you had to give up bread on a ketogenic diet? Just follow this recipe to make your own fat-fuelled loaf that can be used to make sandwiches or even french toast!

Ingredients:
- 1 ½ cup almond flour
- 6 eggs, separated
- 4 tbsp butter, melted
- 3 tsp baking powder
- ¼ tsp cream of tartar
- Pinch of salt

Directions:
1. Preheat oven to 365 degrees Fahrenheit.
2. Add cream of tartar to egg whites, and beat until soft peaks are formed.
3. Combine egg yolks, butter, almond flour, baking powder, and salt in a food processor. Mix until ingredients are combined (The dough will look lumpy).
4. Add ⅓ of egg white mixture to the egg yolk mixture and mix well.

5. Add the remaining ⅔ of the egg white mixture and gently mix until ingredients are well combined. Avoid over mixing to ensure your bread is light and fluffy!
6. Pour mixture into a greased 8x4 loaf pan (or line with baking paper). Bake for 30 minutes.
7. Check bread with a toothpick, which should come out clean.

Enjoy!

Meatloaf Pepper Rings

These mini meatloaf pepper rings are perfect for a fancy dinner gathering or can easily be packed for your lunch at work the next day!

Ingredients:
- 2 bell peppers
- 1 lb ground beef
- 1 egg
- ¼ cup parmesan cheese
- 1 pinch red pepper flakes
- 1 clove garlic, minced
- 1 tbsp olive oil
- 1 tbsp parsley, diced
- 1 large tomato, diced

Directions:
1. Slice the bottoms and the tops from each bell pepper (dice these parts for use in the beef mixture). Then, remove the white lining and seeds. Slice the peppers into three rings, and place on a sheet lined with parchment paper.
2. Then, mix ground beef with egg, parmesan cheese, red pepper flakes, garlic, and diced pepper until well combined.

3. Stuff each pepper ring with beef mixture.
4. Heat olive oil in a frying pan over medium heat. Then, brown each pepper ring for 4-5 minutes on each side.
5. Transfer peppers to baking sheet, and top with diced tomato.
6. Bake for 35-45 minutes.
7. Top with fresh parsley.

Enjoy!

TBLTA (Turkey Bacon, Lettuce, Tomato, Avocado) Wrap

The ultimate comfort food, the traditional BLT gets an upgrade with creamy and delicious avocado!

Ingredients:
- 6 slices turkey bacon, cooked
- 2 lettuce leaves or collard leaves
- ½ tomato, sliced
- 1 avocado, sliced
- 2 tbsp canola-free mayonnaise
- Pinch of pepper

Directions:
1. Lay out lettuce leaves or collard leaves and spread mayonnaise evenly between both wraps.
2. Top wraps with sliced turkey tomato, turkey bacon, and avocado, and add a pinch of pepper.
3. Roll wraps and cut in half.

Enjoy!

Zucchini Noodle with Avocado Pesto Sauce

You can even enjoy pasta (the right way!) on a ketogenic diet. Zucchini noodles are a great replacement for wheat-based pasta, and the creamy pesto sauce is the perfect accoutrement to this fat-fuelled dish.

Ingredients:

- 3 large zucchini
- 2 tbsp olive oil
- 1 avocado
- ½ cup basil leaves
- 2 cloves of garlic, minced
- 3 tbsp pine nuts
- 1 tbsp lemon juice
- Pinch of salt
- Pinch of pepper

Directions:

1. Spiralize your zucchini using a spiralizer or a grater using the largest holes. Place noodles on paper towel so that any excess moisture is absorbed.
2. In a food processor, add avocado, basil leaves, garlic, pine nuts, lemon juice, and sea salt. Pulse until mixture is finely chopped. Then, add 1 tbsp of olive oil slowly until mixture looks creamy.
3. Add 1 tbsp of olive oil in a frying pan over medium heat, and add zucchini noodles. Cook for 1-2 minutes until noodles are tender.
4. Add noodles to a bowl and toss with avocado sauce. Add salt and pepper to taste.

Enjoy!

Garlic Butter Salmon

A simple yet elegant dish that is high in heart-healthy omega-3 fats!

Ingredients:

- 1 ¼ lb sockeye salmon
- 2 tbsp lemon juice
- 2 cloves of garlic, minced
- 2 tbsp butter, cold and cubed
- ½ tsp salt
- Pinch of pepper
- 1 tbsp parsley, chopped

Directions:
1. Preheat oven to 375 degrees Fahrenheit.
2. In a saucepan, combine lemon juice and garlic over medium heat. Add butter and mix gently until butter melts.
3. Place the salmon in a piece of foil. Using a brush or a spoon, brush the salmon with the butter sauce. Add salt and pepper to taste. Cover the salmon with foil, and ensure that all sides are closed so the butter sauce does not leak out.
4. Bake for 12-14 minutes, then remove the foil to allow the salmon to broil for another 2 minutes.
5. Remove the salmon from the oven and top with parsley.

Enjoy!

Coconut Lime Skillet Chicken

If you're craving something a bit more exotic then try this Thai-inspired dish!

Ingredients:
- 4 chicken thighs
- ¼ tsp salt
- Pinch pepper
- 1 tbsp coconut oil
- ½ red onion, chopped

- 1 cup chicken stock
- 1 tbsp lime juice
- ½ tsp red chili flakes
- ½ cup full-fat coconut milk

Directions:
1. Sprinkle chicken thighs with salt and pepper.
2. Melt coconut oil in a large frying pan over medium heat. Add the chicken thighs and cook on each side for 5-7 minutes or until browned. Remove chicken from frying pan and set aside.
3. Add the red onion to the frying pan and saute to soften. Add the chicken stock, lime juice, cilantro, and chili flakes. Bring the mixture to a boil, then reduce to a simmer for five minutes.
4. Add the coconut milk and simmer for another five minutes until mixture has reduced.
5. Add the chicken back to the frying pan, cover, and cook for another 5-10 minutes or until chicken has cooked completely.

Enjoy!

Desserts

Coconut Oil Fudge

You'll be surprised at just how tasty this ketogenic-friendly fudge is without all the added sugar found in traditional versions!

Ingredients:
- 1 cup coconut oil
- 1 cup almond butter
- ¼ cup unsweetened almond milk
- Optional: stevia

Directions:
1. Melt coconut oil in a small saucepan over medium heat. Add almond butter and almond milk and stir until well combined.
2. Pour fudge mixture into a parchment paper lined pan.
3. Refrigerate for two hours, or until set.
4. Cut into slices and serve.

Enjoy!

Blackberry Coconut Fat Bombs

A dessert that is bound the impress, these fat bombs tend to be universally liked by kids and adults alike!

Ingredients:
- 1 cup coconut butter
- 1 cup coconut oil
- ½ cup blackberries
- ½ tsp stevia
- ½ tsp vanilla extract
- 1 tbsp lemon juice

Directions:
1. In a saucepan, combine coconut butter, coconut oil, and blackberries and heat over medium heat until well combined.
2. In a food processor, add saucepan mixture with stevia, vanilla extract, and lemon juice. Process until smooth.
3. Spread mixture in a small parchment paper lined pan.
4. Refrigerate for one hour or until mixture has hardened.
5. Cut into squares and serve!

Enjoy!

Coconut Macaroons

Chewy on the inside, and crisp on the outside. The perfect treat!

Ingredients:

- ¼ cup almond flour
- ½ cup shredded coconut
- ½ tsp stevia
- 1 tsp vanilla extract
- 1 tbsp coconut oil
- 3 egg whites

Directions:

1. Put a medium sized bowl in the fridge in preparation for the egg whites.
2. Preheat oven to 400 degrees Fahrenheit.
3. Mix almond flour and coconut until well combined.
4. Melt coconut oil in a saucepan, and add vanilla extract and stevia.
5. Add the melted coconut oil mixture to the flour mixture and mix until well combined.
6. Put the egg whites in the chilled bowl and whisk until the whites create stiff peaks.
7. Gently combine the egg whites with the flour-oil mixture. Do not overmix.
8. Spoon the mixture onto a parchment paper lined sheet.
9. Bake for 8 minutes or until macaroons appear brown on top.

Enjoy!

Chapter 7: Troubleshooting Guide

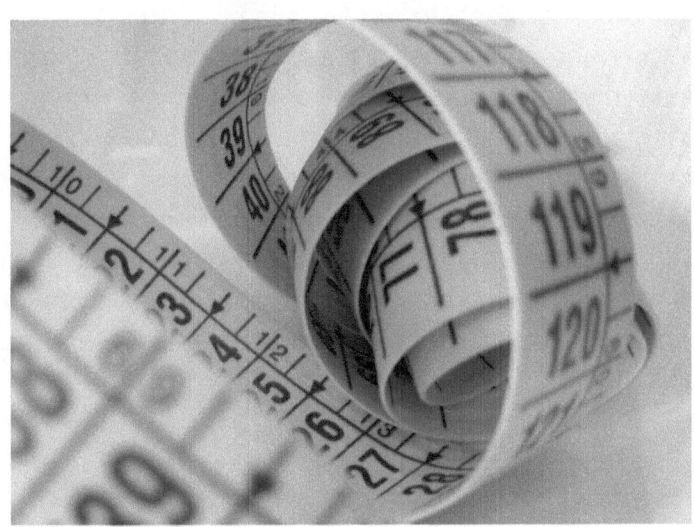

You're excited because you've officially made the switch to a ketogenic diet. You can't wait to start losing weight, think more clearly, and improve your body composition. Unfortunately, it seems that you've hit a few roadblocks and you're not quite sure what to do. Does this mean the ketogenic diet isn't for you? Fortunately, many commonly experienced problems have a simple fix. Just check out this troubleshooting guide below to find the solution for your ketosis conundrum.

Problem #1: Induction Flu (aka 'Keto Flu')

During the initial transition to a ketogenic diet, most people will experience what's commonly known as the 'keto flu'. Symptoms including headaches, fatigue, nausea, brain fog, confusion, and irritability are not uncommon during the first few days to weeks of being on a ketogenic diet.

The Solution: Salt, Water, Fat

Fortunately, these symptoms will disappear by themselves in a few days to a couple weeks by themselves. The main cause of these symptoms is dehydration and lack of salt due to an increase in urination. Therefore, to get over induction flu faster, try drinking more water and adding half a teaspoon of salt to a glass of water to relieve symptoms. You can also drink more broth, which is a hydrating and tasty alternative that will also give you a good dose of sodium. Finally, consider upping your fat intake since many people initially switching to a ketogenic diet don't eat enough. Dieters may be unintentionally under eating after cutting out carbohydrates, which can cause fatigue, irritability and other symptoms. Eating enough healthy fats can speed up the transition and get you over the initial hump.

Problem #2: Leg Cramps

Annoying and sometimes painful, leg cramps can really put a damper on your training schedule or trying to get to sleep at night. Luckily, there are some simple fixes for this problem.

The Solution: Water & Salt, Magnesium, Carbohydrates

Leg cramps are usually the result of a loss of minerals (due to increased urination), so make sure you're drinking enough water and eating enough salt. At the same time, you'll want to replace the magnesium lost due to urination by taking a magnesium supplement. There are a number of different types of magnesium so you may have to experiment with the version that works the best with your body (e.g., citrate, bisglycinate, oxide). As a last resort you could also try increasing your carbohydrates. The caveat is that the more carbohydrates you consume, the fewer benefits you'll experience from being in ketosis all the time.

Problem #3: Constipation

It's hard to feel positive and upbeat if you're chronically constipated. Constipation can be relatively common for those starting a low carbohydrate diet as the digestive system begins to adapt to a higher fat intake.

The Solution: Water & Salt, Fibre, Magnesium

Dehydration is one of the most common causes of constipation, and is a common occurrence on a low-carb diet. The body attempts to relieve your dehydration by absorbing water from the colon, making bowel movements less speedy than they were on a higher carb diet. The best course of action is to ensure you're drinking enough water with a bit of salt to balance your electrolytes. Also, ensure you're getting enough fibre. Some people who start the ketogenic diet are thrilled to be able to eat meat and lard in abundance if they had formerly denied themselves these foods. But your body needs adequate fibre for healthy bowel movements, so make a conscious decision to get enough low-carb vegetables throughout the day including leafy greens, tomatoes, onions, cucumber, and broccoli. Finally, you can also try magnesium since this mineral draws water into the bowels to relieve chronic constipation.

Problem #4: Bad Breath (aka. 'Keto breath')

You would hate for people to think you don't practice good oral hygiene, but fruity or 'fermented' breath is often just a side effect when starting the ketogenic diet.

Solution: Water & Salt, Carbohydrates

'Keto breath' is usually temporary, so if you have the patience to persevere, you'll usually find that your fruity breath returns to normal in a week or two. That being said, drinking more water with a bit of salt can help moisten your mouth, which is needed to wash away odour-producing bacteria. Since ketosis can dehydrate you, you'll likely have to drink more water than you're used to maintain proper hydration. On the other hand, if you can't handle the smell of your breath any longer you could also consider reducing ketosis by eating more carbohydrates. Eating between 50-70g of carbohydrates per day will be enough to take your body out of ketosis, while still giving you the benefits of a low carb diet.

Problem #5: Heart Palpitations

If you've never had them before, heart palpitations can be somewhat fear-provoking. The reason for your these new cardiac irregularities is due to your heart having to pump a bit harder because of reduced blood volume due to dehydration.

Solution: Water, Carbohydrates

The best way to increase blood volume to take the pressure off of your heart is to properly hydrate. So drink up with a bit of salt to restore electrolyte balance and rid yourself of pesky heart palpitations. Heart palpitations usually resolve by themselves within a week or two as the body adjusts to being in ketosis, but if they don't for some reason then you may want to consider increasing your carbohydrate intake. Sometimes heart irregularities can be due to elevated cortisol levels (a stress hormone), which can rise when carbohydrate intake is lowered. If you notice the heart palpitations continue despite being in full ketosis for more than a few weeks than you may want to consider increasing your carbohydrate intake to lower your stress response.

Problem #6: Reduced Athletic Performance

You may notice for the first few weeks on a ketogenic diet that you don't seem to be killing it at the gym like you normally do. Remember, it does take time for your body to become fully fat-adapted so don't expect to become superman or superwoman overnight.

Solution: Water & Salt, Time, Cyclical Ketogenic Dieting

Drinking a large glass of water with half a tsp of salt before a workout will improve your performance while your body is adapting to the diet. Also, remember that it can take up to a few months for your body to become fully adapted to burning fat as fuel instead of sugar, so have patience! That being said, if you are an endurance runner or do other types of aerobic activity then you may perform better on a cyclical ketogenic diet that allows for carb refeeds every 5-6 days. You can plan your performance activities around your refeeds to ensure you'll have adequate liver and muscle glycogen to fuel your activities.

Conclusion

Hopefully this guide has shown you how easy it can be to eat a fat-fueled diet that will help your body shed weight and get fit. Gone are the days where you had to eat bland wholegrain cereal and nonfat milk to be 'healthy'. More and more research is finally demonstrating that fat doesn't make you fat! By eating traditional foods like beef, butter, and coconut, you'll actually be building a better body that has more energy, more lean muscle, and less excess fat! Nutritional ketosis can be a real game changer for many people, so break out the butter and ditch the bread for better health!

If you enjoyed this book or received value from it in any way, then I'd like to ask you for a favor: would you be kind enough to leave a review for this book on Amazon? It'd be greatly appreciated!

References

1.	Nei, M., Ngo, L., Sirven, J. I., & Sperling, M. R. (2014). Ketogenic diet in adolescents and adults with epilepsy. *Seizure, 23*(6), 439-442.

2.	Stewart, W. K., & Fleming, L. W. (1973). Features of a successful therapeutic fast of 382 days' duration. *Postgraduate medical journal, 49*(569), 203-209.

3.	Bueno, N. B., de Melo, I. S. V., de Oliveira, S. L., & da Rocha Ataide, T. (2013). Very-low-carbohydrate ketogenic diet v. low-fat diet for long-term weight loss: a meta-analysis of randomised controlled trials. *British Journal of Nutrition, 110*(07), 1178-1187.

4.	Moreno, B., Crujeiras, A. B., Bellido, D., Sajoux, I., & Casanueva, F. F. (2016). Obesity treatment by very low-calorie-ketogenic diet at two years: reduction in visceral fat and on the burden of disease. *Endocrine, 54*(3), 681-690.

5.	Maalouf, M., Rho, J. M., & Mattson, M. P. (2009). The neuroprotective properties of calorie restriction, the ketogenic diet, and ketone bodies. *Brain research reviews, 59*(2), 293-315.

6.	Gasior, M., Rogawski, M. A., & Hartman, A. L. (2006). Neuroprotective and disease-modifying effects of the ketogenic diet. *Behavioural pharmacology, 17*(5-6), 431.

7.	Yancy, W. S., Olsen, M. K., Guyton, J. R., Bakst, R. P., & Westman, E. C. (2004). A low-carbohydrate, ketogenic diet versus a low-fat diet to treat obesity and hyperlipidemia: a randomized, controlled trial. *Annals of internal medicine, 140*(10), 769-777.

8.	Dashti, H. M., Al-Zaid, N. S., Mathew, T. C., Al-Mousawi, M., Talib, H., Asfar, S. K., & Behbahani, A. I. (2006). Long term effects of ketogenic diet in obese subjects with high cholesterol level. *Molecular and cellular biochemistry, 286*(1-2), 1-9.

9.	Badman, M. K., Kennedy, A. R., Adams, A. C., Pissios, P., & Maratos-Flier, E. (2009). A very low carbohydrate ketogenic diet improves glucose tolerance in ob/ob mice independently of weight loss. *American Journal of Physiology-Endocrinology and Metabolism, 297*(5), E1197-E1204.

10.	Hussain, T. A., Mathew, T. C., Dashti, A. A., Asfar, S., Al-Zaid, N., & Dashti, H. M. (2012). Effect of low-calorie versus low-carbohydrate ketogenic diet in type 2 diabetes. *Nutrition, 28*(10), 1016-1021.

11.	Zhou, W., Mukherjee, P., Kiebish, M. A., Markis, W. T., Mantis, J. G., & Seyfried, T. N. (2007). The calorically restricted ketogenic diet, an effective alternative therapy for malignant brain cancer. *Nutrition & metabolism, 4*(1), 1.

12.	Schmidt, M., Pfetzer, N., Schwab, M., Strauss, I., & Kämmerer, U. (2011). Effects of a ketogenic diet on the quality of life in 16 patients with advanced cancer: A pilot trial. *Nutrition & metabolism, 8*(1), 1.

www.ingramcontent.com/pod-product-compliance
Lightning Source LLC
Chambersburg PA
CBHW050523290526
45786CB00007B/2671